Facing Illness,
Finding Peace

Facing Illness, Finding Peace

By Nancy Groves

auline
BOOKS & MEDIA
Boston

Library of Congress Cataloging-in-Publication Data

Groves, Nancy.
  Facing illness, finding peace / by Nancy Groves. — [Rev. ed.].
       p. cm.
  Rev. ed. of: Faith & illness. 2002.
  ISBN 0-8198-2686-3 (pbk.)
  1. Sick—Religious life.   I. Groves, Nancy. Faith & illness. II. Title.
  BV4910.G76 2009
  248.8'6—dc22

                                                              2009002610

The Scripture quotations contained herein are from the *New Revised Standard Version Bible: Catholic Edition*, copyright © 1989, 1993, Division of Christian Education of the National Council of the Churches of Christ in the United States of America. Used by permission. All rights reserved.

Cover design by Rosana Usselmann

Cover photo by Mary Emmanuel Alves, FSP

Interior photos: Stacie Grange: p. 12; Steve Grange: pp. 4, 84, 116; Patricia Cora Shaules, FSP: p. 94; Mary Domenica Vitello, FSP: pp. xiii, 125

"P" and PAULINE are registered trademarks of the Daughters of St. Paul.

Published by Pauline Books & Media, 50 Saint Paul's Avenue, Boston, MA 02130-3491

Printed in the U.S.A.

www.pauline.org

Pauline Books & Media is the publishing house of the Daughters of St. Paul, an international congregation of women religious serving the Church with the communications media.

1 2 3 4 5 6 7 8 9   13 12 11 10 09

In memory of
Donald Groves,
whose spirit of love
remains with us forever

———❦———

Dedicated to
Katherine Groves,
whose life embraces
her father's joy

CONTENTS

INTRODUCTION

The crisis of ill health affects us all
at some time in our lives.
For many of us, the duration is short,
and recovery is soon.

However, there are others who must
confront the crisis of a chronic
progressive disease, or
a life-threatening illness, and this
reality may be a continuing part of life.

The onset of the disease may come
at any age, making the road
ahead one filled with fears,
apprehensions, and anxieties.

Too often, it feels as if the road is traveled alone.

And yet, from the beginning of this journey,
the still and gentle voice of Jesus asks us
if we will allow him to walk with us.
And so we choose love over fear,
and Jesus becomes our blessed companion
on this road.

As you walk with him, this book
will be your companion

— A guide to understanding the
emotional impact of facing a serious illness;

— An instrument that
encourages you to share your thoughts
with a friend, family member, priest,
or minister;

— A source of comfort for
the days when your heart
is weary from the struggle;

— A help to heighten your awareness
of your uniqueness and beauty
that no disease can touch or change;

— A reminder of Jesus' everlasting love.

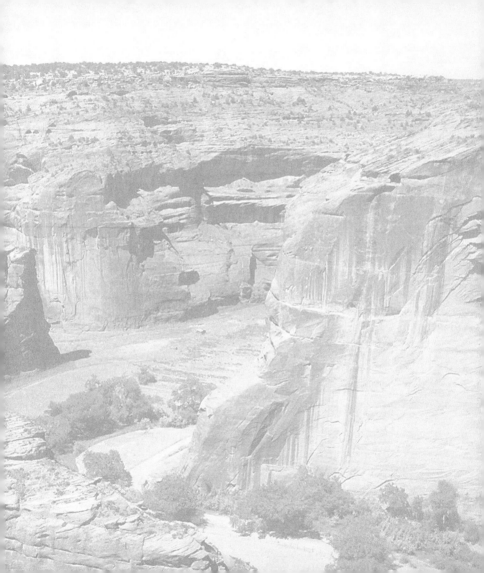

SOMETHING'S WRONG: SEARCHING FOR AN ANSWER

Surely God is my salvation;
I will trust, and will not be afraid,
for the LORD GOD is my strength
and my might; he has become my
salvation.

ISAIAH 12:2

How many days or months have
passed with the recurring
feelings of fatigue and discomfort,
and of having a sense that all is
not right within?

The internal messages are
constant, yet subtle,
reminding me of storm clouds
ominously forming in the skies.

I am left to wonder when
the storm
    will
        appear.

I feel helpless and
frightened.

My doctor is concerned.
His face mirrors my
apprehensions. He
cannot diagnose the
problem until more tests
are done. I am tired of
subjecting my body
to the invasions of strange
tubes and X-rays.

I am becoming an illness
to be diagnosed
instead of a person
who is suffering.

See me.
    See *me* please!

It is over. The illness
has been named. I am
part of a national
average—a statistic—
and I am sometimes
referred to as my disease.

That only increases my pain.

It is over.
    The illness has been named.

It is over—
    or is this only the
        beginning for
            me?

Reflections

Knowing the disease I must face brings new concerns to me. What do I need to know about my illness?

Has the knowledge of this illness changed my priorities in life?

What is most important to me now?

Prayer

Dear God, I am frightened. I wanted an answer. Now I have received one, and I am afraid. I want this to be a bad dream that will end when I awaken to tomorrow's sunlight. But tomorrow's arrival will not erase the reality of today. Stay close, dear Father, and let me feel the warmth of your Son's light on me as I face today ... and tomorrow. Amen.

*Do not let your hearts be troubled,
and do not let them be afraid.*

JOHN 14:27

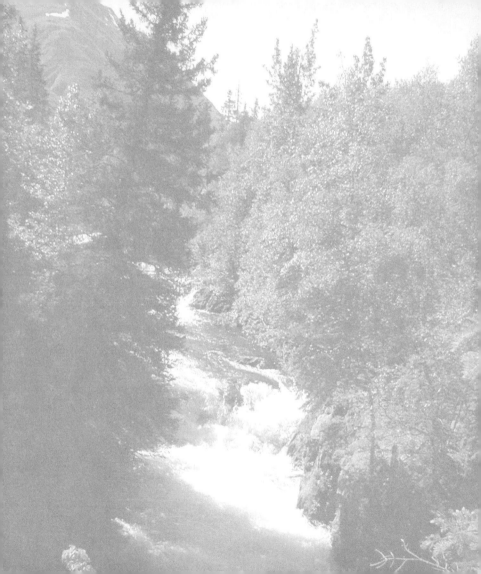

WHAT AM I FEELING?

SHOCK

ANXIETY

ANGER

DEPRESSION

GUILT

SHAME

Turn to me and be gracious to me,
for I am lonely and afflicted.
Relieve the troubles of my heart,
and bring me out of my distress.

PSALM 25:16–17

SHOCK

Sad

Hurt

Outraged

Confused

bro**K**en

Trust in him at all times ...
pour out your heart before him;
God is a refuge for us.

PSALM 62:8

I know now what I must face.
The cause of my apprehensions
has been named. But the future
is still filled with unknowns.
The uncertainties frighten me.

What am I feeling?

What makes that question
so difficult to answer?

It is as though my body
is not my own, as though
a stranger has invaded my
frame. I feel cut off from
my emotions.

I am numb, overwhelmed,
afraid I will be unable to
cope. I can't face it—
not yet. I don't want to
discuss it, for then it
becomes too real
    for me.

I want life to continue on
as before. Talk with
me about the news, the
weather, the latest fashions,
    anything but sickness.

Don't look at me with
sadness in your eyes,
or sympathy,
    or fear.
That only shows me the
pain I have brought to
you. I can't deal with
that now.

I need some distance
from this new reality.

Let me find comfort
in ignoring this—
in denying this—
if I must.

Denial is my refuge.

Allow me that.

Reflections

What was my immediate reaction to the news
of my illness?

How did that reaction help me to cope
with this news?

Reflections

What is my reaction to my illness now? How is it different?

How can my faith in God help me in this crisis?

Prayer

Dear Jesus, I thought I was strong, but I am not. I thought I could face this, but I cannot. I thought I could handle anything—I was wrong. Instead, I hide from this frightening reality. In my solitude, I hear you calling out to me—to bring me back to the fold of your love. I cannot hide from you, dear Jesus; you are always with me. Your presence enters my thoughts and my heart. The strength of your love sustains me in the midst of this inner turmoil. You are my refuge. Amen.

As the Father has loved me, so
I have loved you; abide in my love.

JOHN 15:9

ANXIETY

Apprehensive

Nervous

e**X**hausted

Insecure

Empty

Tense

uneas**Y**

Cast all your anxiety on him,
because he cares for you.

1 PETER 5:7

Feelings of apprehension
are beginning to surface.
At times, the anxiety seems
    immobilizing.

How can I unlock its grip?

Perhaps I need to examine
these feelings more closely.
I ask myself …
What brings this anxiety?

Just asking the question
frees me to discover
the answer.

The source is fear.

I am afraid of the
uncertainties that lie ahead.

I am afraid of loneliness—
afraid that my illness will
keep others away.

I am afraid of the pain
and sorrow I may have
to endure.

I am afraid
   of losing control,
   of losing my abilities,
   of losing parts of my body,
      of losing myself.

My awareness of these fears lessens the anxiety for me. It does not remove the anxiety from my life, but it seems to make it less overwhelming and more manageable.

I have learned that being afraid is okay. I realize there is a purpose to my fears. They give me opportunities to grow beyond them.

Sharing my fears is the
next step for me.
Keeping them within
brings emotional isolation
and depression.

Finding someone to listen
may not be easy. I know
my illness can trigger many
fears in others, making
avoidance easier for them.

But I must approach
others and invite them
into my life. I must take
care of myself and teach
others what I need
from them.

Those
who are open to me,
who love me, and
who are willing to learn
will take away the fears
and be my refuge
in this time of need.

How precious they
are to me.

Reflections

What fears am I experiencing as a result of this illness?

Are these fears helping me? What would lessen them for me?

(For Catholics) Is now perhaps the time for me to ask for the sacrament of the Anointing of the Sick, to receive the grace the Lord wants to give me?

Prayer

Dear Jesus, there is a comfort in bringing my fears to you, for I know that your perfect love is greater than all the anxieties of this world. I hear your gentle wisdom in the words of my loved ones who respond to my apprehensions. I call your name, and your voice brings me to a place of tranquility once again. Through your loving compassion, I feel your peace abiding within me. Amen.

I sought the LORD, and he answered me,
and delivered me from all my fears.

PSALM 34:4

ANGER

Annoyed

e**N**raged

Guilty

Exasperated

Regretful

Cast your burden on the LORD,
and he will sustain you . . .

PSALMS 55:22

These last few days have been
increasingly difficult for me.
I seem to lash out at others for
no apparent reason.

I am negative and sarcastic
to people who are trying to
be kind and understanding.

What is going on within me?

I am told I seem angry. Can
I admit to feeling angry?

Anger isn't always
understood or accepted.
It usually scares people
away and causes others
to be critical and judgmental.

And yet,
    I AM ANGRY.

I am angry that I have been
afflicted with this illness.

I am angry that I must be
dependent on others.

I am angry that I have
been relieved of responsibilities
that I am still able to assume.

I am angry that people
treat me differently now.

I am angry that I am
losing control over my
life.

I AM ANGRY
    and
I feel guilty because of
    my anger.

It is okay to be angry—

    I am human.

Since my bed is oftentimes
my only companion in
the day, I have learned to
deal with my anger there.

Beating pillows is one of
my pastimes. It's my way of
trying to get rid of anger that
might otherwise keep loved
ones away.

Even better is sharing my anger
with God, a listener who
accepts me where
I am and who
tells me ...
    he can handle it.

Yes,
    I am angry
        and
    I accept where I am
        and
    I can handle it ... now.

IT IS OKAY TO BE ANGRY ...
    I AM HUMAN.

Reflections

How do I show my anger?

Can I accept anger as being a normal and understandable reaction to my illness?

Can I be honest about my anger? Can I even admit that I am angry with God?

Prayer

Dear God, it is hard for me to admit it, but not only am I angry, I am angry at you. I feel angry that illness has come to me—this kind, at this time, in this way. I feel like yelling, "Why did you do this to me?" At the same time, I am relieved that I am able to say this to you. This honest expression of my anger allows me to examine my faith with greater depth and clarity. So I bring my anger to you, and in doing so, open my heart to your love and understanding. Amen.

Trust in him at all times, O people;
pour out your heart before him …

Psalm 62:8

DEPRESSION

Despondent

Empty

Powerless

Regretful

Exasperated

Sorrowful

Solemn

Isolated

Overwhelmed

Numb

Surely he has borne our
infirmities and carried our diseases …

ISAIAH 53:4

I don't think I can face today.

I have no energy to leave this
bed or to talk with anyone.
I seem to be in a place
I've not been before.

I feel hopeless.

There seems to be no
reason to continue with
my life. I can't control
my tears. They are endless
as they stream down my face
and fall into my empty hands.

Isn't my life, too, empty—
void of meaning and
purpose?

I have lost my valiant
fight with this illness.

I have no strength to go on.

My loved ones seem
frightened of my sorrow.
They bring me gifts, shower
me with flowers to
    "cheer me up."

They are constantly
doing something
for me …

> straightening my
>   sheets
> fluffing my
>   pillows
> opening my
>   drapes
> reading my
>   get well cards
> bringing my
>   food.

I wonder if they are doing
these things to avoid the
emotional discomfort my
illness brings.

Their acts of kindness
do not go unnoticed,
although I am unable to
convey any appreciation.

The sorrow and the
emptiness remain.

In the midst of these
caring people, scurrying
to do something to lift
my spirits, I feel
    isolated
        and
            alone.

I feel no comfort.

Then you enter my room.
You see my tears.
My sadness frightens
you. Your face searches
mine for an answer …

I have none to give you.

You draw near to me, place
your arms around me, and I
rest my head upon your shoulder.
I hold you close. My tears fall.
We do not speak. And yet, your
presence tells me of your love
and compassion.

Your gift to me is
yourself, your
honest,
    silent, and beautiful
        expression of
            compassion.

Your gift of presence
relieves my feelings
of isolation and despair.

While others are
doing for me,
    you are
        being with me.

That is what I need right now.
That is what comforts my soul.

Thank you
for being in my life.

Today, you shared my
pain and sadness.

Tomorrow will be a better day.

I think I can face
tomorrow
all because
of you.

Reflections

What makes this illness most difficult for me?

What comforts me when I feel hopeless and in despair?

How does my faith bring comfort to me?

Prayer

Dear Jesus, the sadness I am feeling extends beyond my physical body and touches my soul. I feel so distant from your love ... so alone with this illness. Alone—as you were in the Garden of Gethsemane; abandoned by sleeping disciples; forgotten in your darkest hour. In my own moments of despair, I cry out to you in prayer, asking for a sign of your presence. And you do not forsake me, but answer in the form of a beloved friend whose care and physical embrace carry your love to my soul. Amen.

For just as the sufferings of Christ are abundant for us, so also our consolation is abundant through Christ.

2 Corinthians 1:5

GUILT

Grieved

Upset

Inadequate

Loathsome

Troubled

[L]et them return to the LORD,
that he may have mercy on them,
and to our God, for he will
abundantly pardon.

ISAIAH 55:7

I need to find a reason for this illness.

I ask myself
    over and
        over again,
            Why Me?

In my search for an answer,
I remember past behaviors
that ...
    may have offended
    may have caused pain
    may have been unjust
        uncalled for
        egotistical
        arrogant
        foolish
        selfish
        cruel.

The list of possibilities mounts
as does my guilt.
Is this illness a form of
retribution for past sins?
Is my illness the price I
must pay?

Something deep within
me stirs and
answers … no.

God gently reminds me
that this illness is
not a punishment for sin.

There is no answer to
my question—
    Why Me?

Disease and suffering
do not come from God.

Rather, illness is part of the
mystery of human life
on this earth.

It is a consequence of
    being human.

I cannot search for
logic or justice.
Life is not logical
    or fair.

Life simply is.

As I look back on my
life, I have regrets …
words I wish I had not said.
   Things I wish I had not done.

The past cannot be changed,
but I might need to ask for
and receive
forgiveness from others.

Still, that is not enough
to remove the pain of my self-reproach.
My sins affect not only
my relationships with others, but also
my relationship with God.

I must search my heart and,
in contrition, ask God for
forgiveness.

Mercy and forgiveness
are the gifts God
most loves to give.

As I am touched with God's
mercy, the burden is lifted.
The guilt is gone.

Reflections

What are my past sins that burden my heart?

Do I need to make amends to others?

(For Catholics) Do I realize the great gift that is offered in the sacrament of Reconciliation (also called confession)? Is now the time to ask for this gift?

What is my response to God's mercy and forgiveness?

Prayer

Dear Father, I come to you to ask forgiveness for all the ways I have failed to live according to your will for me, and out of love for you and others. Your gifts to me were not only for me, but so that I could make the world a better place. I'm sorry for the times I used my gifts selfishly instead of generously. Help me to live now as a person of peace and reconciliation, sharing with others the peace and forgiveness that you have given me. Amen.

All this is from God, who reconciled us to himself through Christ, and has given us the ministry of reconciliation.

2 CORINTHIANS 5:18

SHAME

Sad
Humiliated
Angry
Miserable
Embarrassed

*… I will not be put to shame in
any way, but … with all boldness,
Christ will be exalted now as always
in my body …*

PHILIPPIANS 1:20

My self-sufficiency is waning.
I am embarrassed that I need others
to help me with everyday tasks.

Waiting for others to
assist me is not easy.
It is not that I am impatient.
Waiting just reminds me
of my inabilities.

I used to be such a
private person.
I enjoyed my time alone
    to bathe,
        groom, and
        dress myself.

Those precious moments
are too few now.

So many of the things I used to
do for myself are now being
done to me or for me. If I must accept
this—as part of my illness—
then I must identify what I need
from others to lessen the
    shame I am feeling.

I have made a list of what I need.

If I can receive these things,
I will have within my grasp
what I so
    desperately need ...
        self-respect
        and dignity.

Speak to me, not about me, when I am in your
presence.

Enjoy my company. Laugh with me.

Listen to me when I speak with you.

Forgive my anger if I lose patience with myself.

Respect my need for privacy.

Enable me to keep my feelings of worth.

Show me your love and compassion.

Place items I need within reach of my hands.

Enter my room after you have knocked.

Cry with me. Sorrow shared brings emotional
comfort.

Treat me as a valued human being, despite my
disfigurement or disability.

Reflections

What situations bring feelings of shame?

What do I need from others to lessen the shame that I feel?

Many people were brought to Jesus who felt ashamed because of their afflictions. How did Jesus respond to them?

How does reflecting on Christ's compassion relieve my sense of shame?

Prayer

Dear God, there are no feelings of shame or embarrassment when I speak with you. You remind me that in spite of my limitations, the essence of who I am will never change. My worth is not measured by what I am able to do. I am worthy because I was created by you and because I am loved by you. Thank you for the growth in freedom that I am experiencing as I learn to let go and surrender to your love. Amen.

O guard my life, and deliver me; do not let me be put to shame, for I take refuge in you.

PSALM 25:20

ADJUSTING TO ENDLESS CHANGES

God is our refuge and strength,
a very present help in trouble.

PSALMS 46:1

There have been so many
changes since this disease
entered my body.

Some of
    my abilities have
        changed to inabilities
    my strengths to fears
    my self-assurances
        to self-doubts.

Responding to these changes
is not easy. In the process of
trying to adjust to this
disease, I have lost so much.

I have lost my independence.
I am no longer self-sufficient.

I have lost my sense of
security. I have so many
questions about my future.

How will this disease progress?
Who will care for me?
Are my finances adequate to
meet my medical needs?

I have lost my ability to complete
plans. The unfinished projects
remind me of skills I may never
be able to use again.

I have lost my dreams and my
hopes. A carefree future filled
with travel and comfort is no
longer a realistic goal.

I have lost some friends who
find it too painful to remain
in my life. My illness reminds
them of their own
    vulnerabilities
        to disease.

I have lost aspects of myself
and my identity. My physical
body has changed, as
    have my abilities.

With this loss of appearance
    and loss of function,
        I feel a loss
          of self.

These losses grieve me,
    and I mourn them.

As I confront these losses,
I am in touch with an increasing
sense of losing control.

I feel angry because I have
    lost control over my life.

Without control,
    I feel
        powerless
        hopeless
        dependent
        ineffective
        helpless
        inadequate.

Hospital stays are most
distressing to me. It is
there that I lose the sense
of who I am.

My identity fades as I take
part in my new role
   of patient.

My thoughts, feelings,
and preferences are lost
in the medical regimen I
am told I must follow.

I am given no opportunity to
decide what will be done for me
or when it will occur.
The hospital routines add to
my sense of isolation.
To many of the medical staff,
I am ...
> an entity without rights,
> a disease to be treated.

And in response, I feel
> powerless
> hopeless
> dependent
> ineffective
> helpless
> inadequate.

I feel a loss of control.

Being hospitalized and receiving
treatments helps control my
pain and the progression
    of this disease.

For that, I am grateful.

But the emotional price
I pay is great. It is only when
I return home, where I am more
in control of my environment
and myself, that I begin to feel
better about
    who I am.

Being home has its own set
of adjustments. It is here
that I interact with loved ones.

Sometimes, the struggle
seems greater for my loved ones.
They share their feelings
of helplessness as they search
for ways to help me adjust
to this disease.

Learning about the illness and the
path of progression to expect
helps us to adjust, for this
lessens some of the
uncertainties that are a
part of the future.

Teaching my loved ones
how to care for me, when
needed, lessens their feelings
of helplessness and provides
them with something
important to do.

I try to impress upon them,
that while their actions
help me, it is
    their loving presence
        that heals me.

I don't think I could
cope with this illness
    without feeling
        their love.

There is grief for my loved
ones. They, too, have
lost many things.

They have lost a healthy
person in their life
who was needed for
emotional and
    financial security.

They have lost someone
who was always busy,
maintaining the home,
caring for the children.

They have lost the plans
for retirement years.

They have lost the dreams
for a future where
    illness plays no part.

They have lost the comfort
    of their regular
        daily routine.

The whole family situation
is changing. Things I can no
longer do are being
        done by others.

Responsibilities shift,
tasks change, emotions rise.

There is anger and resentment.

Someone feels burdened with
the changes that are occurring.
The stability that once existed
    is now gone.

Home is no longer a refuge
from the outside pressures
of life. Home is now a
source of pressure
    because of my illness.

There is guilt
    because of the anger.

There are questions. How can
anger be justified when a loved
one is ill? But I understand the
frustrations and the emotional
and physical depletion my loved ones
are experiencing
    because of my illness.

Anger is okay.
    Guilt is not necessary.

There is sorrow because of
the losses they are experiencing.

There is hopelessness,
    for there may be no cure
    or chance for recovery.

There is a longing to return
    to the world of yesterday
    when there was
        peace
        comfort
        stability
        health.

My illness is not only within
me. The disease spreads to
all my loved ones and causes
them anguish.

I feel I am a burden.

I wish I could change things
so that life would be easier
    for those I love.

I cannot.

Therein lies my deepest sadness.
        I love them so.

Reflections

What are some of the adjustments I have had to
make because of this illness? Which are the
most difficult?

What has helped me make these changes?

Where can I see the never-changing love of
God at work in my life?

Reflections

How is my illness affecting my loved ones?

How can I help them as they try to adjust to my illness?

Has anything remained constant for me or for my loved ones?

Prayer

Dear Jesus, I do not know which is more difficult for me—adjusting to this illness or seeing the hardships my loved ones must endure. You must have felt like this as you watched your mother at the foot of your cross, suffering because of your suffering. I have struggled to ease their burdens, but my attempts have been in vain. So, I come to you, and I place my family in your outstretched arms, confident that you will heal their heartache and bring them peace. Amen.

> *[H]e raises up the needy out of distress, and makes their families like flocks.... Let them thank the Lord for his steadfast love....*
>
> Psalm 107:41, 31

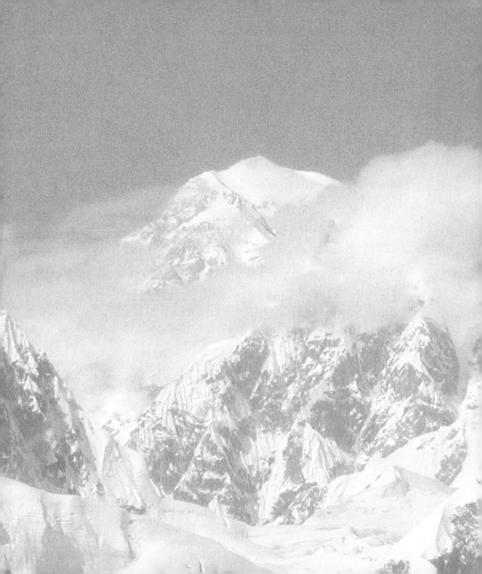

SURVIVAL

So we do not lose heart.
Even though our outer nature
is wasting away,
our inner nature is being renewed
day by day.

2 CORINTHIANS 4:16

Life is becoming a
constant struggle.
I exist from day
    to day.
I search for meaning
in my life
    and find none.

I am not needed
    as I was before.
I cannot perform
    as I did before.
I am beginning to question
    who I am,
    the purpose of my existence.

I look in the mirror
   only to see a stranger there.

What has become
   of my life?

What has become
   of me?

I think of all that
I am going through—
      the treatments that I once
      hoped would cure me.

How much longer
can I endure them?

I know that ending medical
treatment and letting the
disease take its course
is an option.

At times, it seems to
be the logical answer,
    for I feel as though
    I am steadily
        dying.

Why prolong the
    process?

Indeed, why not hasten it?

Thoughts of death
    enter my mind.
Temptations to suicide.

Is that possibly the answer
    to the anguish
        I am feeling?
    To the pain
    I am bringing
        to my loved ones?

Or will my death
only hurt them more?

I have allowed this disease
to do more than affect me
    physically.

I have allowed it to affect
    my thoughts,
        my feelings,
            my reason
            for being.

I have allowed it to take
away all meaning
    in my life.

If I allow this to continue,
  I have no chance
    of survival.

Perhaps the time will come when
  my treatments are
  no longer effective,
and instead
  impose more pain and confusion
  on moments meant to be cherished.

But I must decide now…

Will I choose to live?
The decision must be made,
  and it must be made
    NOW.

  I choose life.

Reflections

How long have I lived with this illness?

Have treatments become too burdensome to me, compared with the potential for good they bring?

How has this illness affected my thoughts and my reason for living?

What do I need from myself and from others to help me choose life?

Prayer

Dear Jesus, I believe in the preciousness of life. It is your gift, and only you may decide when it will end. But lately, I have felt the yearning to return home to you and to leave this earthly body behind. Please surround me with your loving presence, so that I will have the patience to wait until you call me home, and the wisdom to use well the time I have left. Amen.

[M]y desire is to depart and be with Christ, for that is far better; but to remain in the flesh is more necessary for you.

PHILIPPIANS 1:23–24

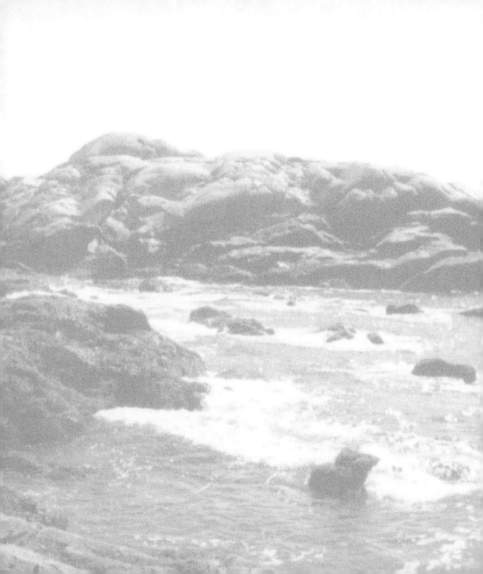

HEALING

I have called you by name,
you are mine ... you are
precious in my sight, and
honored, and I love you.

ISAIAH 43:1, 4

I choose to live and
I choose to live
    with meaning
        and
        purpose.

Who am I?

Am I defined
    by my appearance,
    by my abilities?

Do I really want to limit
the meaning of who I am
    to just two aspects
        of myself?

What else makes me
who I am?

I have many qualities.

Within me lie—
  sensitivity
  compassion
  gentleness
  kindness
  understanding
  caring
  humor
  love
  joy
  creativity
  wisdom
  affection
  honesty
  fairness
  forgiveness and
  a deep devotion to God.

These qualities remain
in spite
of my disease.

I have grown in these virtues
over my lifetime, and I have
new opportunities to grow in them
every day.

As I reflect on these virtues,
another profound realization enters my heart.
Jesus reminds me that I am loved
simply because I am.

Knowing this
gives me inner strength,
rekindles my feelings of worth,
and restores a feeling of hope
for the future.

Life takes on a new meaning.

I am beginning to see myself
in a new light.

Facing this crisis has given me
increased sensitivity and
awareness, and has
strengthened my faith.

The self-doubts have changed
to renewed confidence.

The inabilities have evolved
    into new and
    different skills.

The change in my physical
appearance has led to
    an awareness of
    the beauty that has
      always existed
      within me and
    an awareness of my
    spiritual essence that
      is unchanging.

When this disease first
entered my body, I struggled
to understand the message
    it brought to my life.

Now, I realize it is I
who must decide what
    that message will be.

It is I who must give this
disease a meaning
        in my life.

My reactions to this illness
    determine that meaning.

If I choose to respond with
bitterness and anger,
    then I become
    a bitter and angry person.

If I choose to respond with
    an acceptance of the
    unfairness of my suffering
    and with a determination to
    live fully
        in spite of my illness,
        then
        I open my life to
        God's grace and to
        limitless possibilities
        for new growth.

As I humbly reflect on
the suffering and death of Jesus,
I realize that love is what gave
meaning to his suffering.
  Union with his redemptive love
  is a gift offered to all.

As I embrace Christ's redeeming love,
I am able to strengthen my capacities for
    patience
    forgiveness
    cheerfulness
    insight
    love
    and becoming the person Jesus would
      have me be.

And I can begin to accept with love,
although I do not understand,
the suffering that this illness brings.

Tomorrow is a new day.
A day filled with
    opportunities
    challenges
    hopes and
    dreams.

The fear of tomorrow
        is gone.
The pain of yesterday
        is lessened.

The strength, the love,
    and the acceptance
    of who I am
        make today
        a more beautiful day.

Reflections

Has this illness changed my outlook on life?
If so, in what way?

How will I choose to respond to my illness?
What meaning will I give this illness in my life?

What gifts of grace did I experience as I joined
my suffering with the suffering of Christ?

Reflections

What inner qualities have remained a part of me
in spite of this illness?

What Christ-like qualities do I want to nurture
in myself?

Am I truly convinced that I am a special and
worthwhile person, a beloved child of God?

Prayer

Dear Jesus, I reflect on the redemptive gift of your suffering, and I am humbled by the magnitude and depth of your love. Being loved by you is a truth that lifts my spirit to new heights. I am no longer my disease. I am a child of God, loved completely for who I am. In that love, I find consolation, strength, and inner peace. Amen.

[B]y his wounds, you have been healed.

1 PETER 2:24

PEACE

Those of steadfast mind you keep
in peace—
in peace because they trust in
you.

ISAIAH 26:3

Many days have passed
now, and while my future
remains uncertain, there
exists within me
　　a peacefulness from God
　　that enables me
　　to live
　　　　meaningfully,
　　　　joyously, and
　　　　fully.

There are still days
of rain—
    days of physical pain
    and emotional discomfort.

And on those days, I have
learned to look toward my faith
in God's love, which is
    a sun that shines
    within myself,
    within others.
For when I do, a rainbow
fills my thoughts,
    giving me the
    inner peace
        and healing
           I need.

I am in a different place now.
I have struggled with this
illness and I have found
    some answers
      for my life.

I accept life as it is.
I give thanks for God's love
    that surrounds me.
I look to the possibilities
    and opportunities
    of each day and
I rejoice in the knowledge
    of who I am.

I am a worthwhile, unique, and
　　beautiful person made in God's image.
No matter what life brings to me,
　　God's love for me,
　　my worth,
　　my uniqueness, and
　　my beauty
　　　　will never change.

Therein lies my peace.

Reflections

As I have faced this illness, how have
I experienced the gift of God's peace?

What Scriptures bring peace to my mind
and soul?

In this moment of peace, what do I want to
remember for the times when fear and doubt
may resurface?

Prayer

Dear Father, your love has taught me that inner peace is not found in my external world. Instead, it is a gift that comes through trust in you. I can always return to find it deep within me. I can find that place of tranquility by turning my thoughts to you and resting in the knowledge that you are always with me. Amen.

And the peace of God, which surpasses all understanding, will guard your hearts and your minds in Christ Jesus.

PHILIPPIANS 4:7

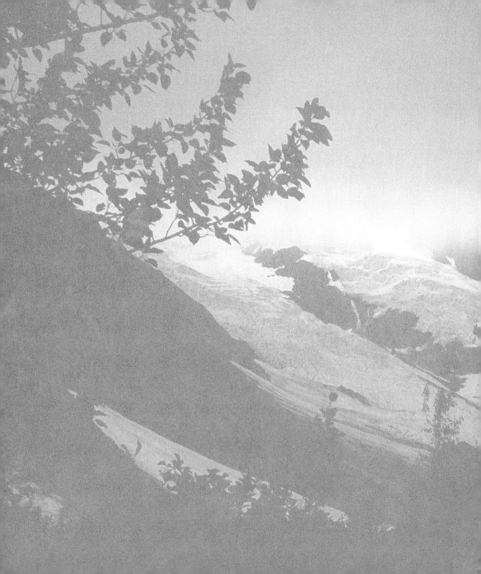

GOD'S GIFT OF HEALING

*For I am convinced that neither
death, nor life ... nor anything else
in all creation, will be able to
separate us from the love of God in
Christ Jesus our Lord.*

ROMANS 8:38–39

*[R]emember, I am with you always,
to the end of the age.*

MATTHEW 28:20

God has been patient with me
during this illness.

When I was angry,
he did not turn away.

When I was filled with despair,
he sent his compassion in the
arms of those who held me.

When I was filled with guilt
and remorse,
he gently whispered his
forgiveness in my heart.

When I was ashamed of the
changes in my body, he reminded
me that I was made in his image,
with an inner beauty
that was eternal.

When I was bitter and called
him unjust and cruel,
he listened and remained
constant in his love.

When my heart was breaking
for my loved ones, he
encompassed them in the circle
of his love and brought them
comfort and strength.

When I found a renewed
meaning in my life, in spite
of my illness, he shared my joy.

My path has never been
traveled alone.
Throughout this experience,
God has offered the gentle
warmth of his constant love.

Now, I bask in the glow of
his love, and I feel the healing
power of his compassion.
Death is no longer an enemy
to be feared. It is, instead,
the final path to my home
with God.

My friends and loved ones
   pray for my body to heal.
They do not understand that
   my healed body may take
   the form of
      a resurrected body.

For is not true healing found
   in the glory of the resurrection?

When my time comes to leave
   this earthly home, I hope the
   memories of moments shared
   will help heal the sense of loss
   for my loved ones.

Memories are a gift from
    God to those left behind.

They bring comfort, joy,
    and laughter, and they
    enable me to live forever
    in the hearts of those I love.

Until we meet again.

*"Do not let not your hearts be troubled.
Believe in God, believe also in me. In my
Father's house are many dwelling-places.
If it were not so, would I have told
you that I go and prepare a place
for you? I will come again and
will take you to myself, so that where I
am, there you may be also...
I am the way, and the truth, and the life."*

JOHN 14:1–3, 6

Prayer

Dear Father, may your love bring peace and comfort to my loved ones, and as for me, may I rest in your arms. Amen.

About the Author

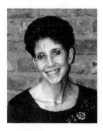

Nancy Groves, MSW, CSW, is a medical social worker with over twenty years of experience as an educator and counselor. She has presented many seminars in hospital, university, and church settings on the emotional impact of serious illness, and she has served on the Michigan Department of Public Health AIDS Advisory Board.

Other helpful reading ...

Surviving Depression
A Catholic Approach
Kathryn J. Hermes, FSP

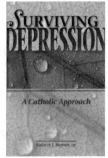

Depression can strike anyone, even those deeply committed to living the Christian life. This reassuring book includes: encouraging stories of others who have lived with depression; psychological, medical, spiritual, and practical self-care perspectives; tips for friends and family of the depressed.

    0-8198-7077-3
    $12.95

The Surviving Depression Journal
A CatholicApproach
Kathryn J. Hermes, FSP

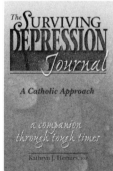

This companion to the best-selling book, *Surviving Depression,* creates a safe space in which people can journal their struggles and fears and come to a deeper sense of hope, peace, and trust.

    0-8198-7104-4
    $12.95

Prayers for Surviving Depression
Kathryn J. Hermes, FSP

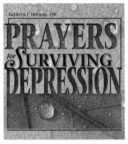

This unique prayer book offers prayers from those who have suffered through depression and yet continue to search for light and strength in their faith. Together with favorite prayers from the Catholic tradition, they offer comfort and hope that God is close to the brokenhearted.

0-8198-5952-4
$10.95

Making Peace with Yourself
15 Steps to Spiritual Healing
Kathryn J. Hermes, FSP

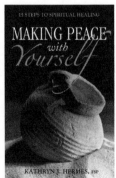

An essential guide to making peace with life as it is, and finding the face of God in the midst of life's confusion. Poignant and touching real-life narratives offer hope and direction.

0-8198-4859-X
$12.95

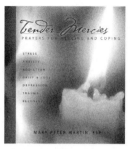

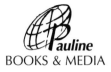

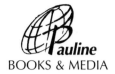

BOOKS & MEDIA

The Daughters of St. Paul operate book and media centers at the following addresses. Visit, call or write the one nearest you today, or find us on the World Wide Web, www.pauline.org.

CALIFORNIA
3908 Sepulveda Blvd, Culver City, CA 90230   310-397-8676
2640 Broadway Street, Redwood City, CA 94063   650-369-4230
5945 Balboa Avenue, San Diego, CA 92111   858-565-9181

FLORIDA
145 S.W. 107th Avenue, Miami, FL 33174   305-559-6715

HAWAII
1143 Bishop Street, Honolulu, HI 96813   808-521-2731
Neighbor Islands call: 866-521-2731

ILLINOIS
172 North Michigan Avenue, Chicago, IL 60601   312-346-4228

LOUISIANA
4403 Veterans Memorial Blvd, Metairie, LA 70006   504-887-7631

MASSACHUSETTS
885 Providence Hwy, Dedham, MA 02026   781-326-5385

MISSOURI
9804 Watson Road, St. Louis, MO 63126   314-965-3512

NEW JERSEY
561 U.S. Route 1, Wick Plaza, Edison, NJ 08817   732-572-1200

NEW YORK
150 East 52nd Street, New York, NY 10022   212-754-1110

PENNSYLVANIA
9171-A Roosevelt Blvd, Philadelphia, PA 19114   215-676-9494

SOUTH CAROLINA
243 King Street, Charleston, SC 29401   843-577-0175

VIRGINIA
1025 King Street, Alexandria, VA 22314   703-549-3806

CANADA
3022 Dufferin Street, Toronto, ON M6B 3T5   416-781-9131

¡También somos su fuente para libros,
videos y música en español!